GAGA OVER

YO

C000127358

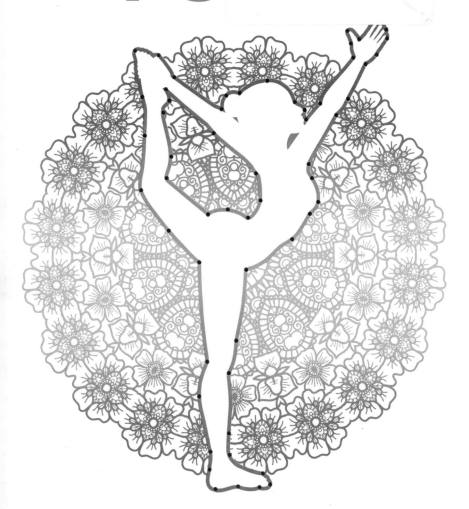

First edition 2017
Offshoot Books
An imprint of Kalabindu Enterprises Pvt. Ltd

GF–18, Virat Bhavan
Commercial Complex, Mukherjee Nagar
Delhi 110009
Phone: +91-11-47038000 / Fax: +91-11-
47038099
Website: www.offshootbooks.com

Dear Reader,

Thank you for buying this book. We hope you enjoy every page of the book—and while you do that, please ensure that no one uses or transmits any part of this publication,
in any form or by any means, without our prior written permission. You wouldn't want to offend the no-offence brand.

In case we haven't mentioned it before, we truly think that you are our favorite reader. Thanks for being a part of the Offshoot universe.

Have fun!

Love,
Team Offshoot

ISBN: 978-93-86362-37-7
Printed in India
Picture credits: www.shutterstock.com

MEANING OF
YOGA

Yoga is not as boring as it sounds. The word comes from the Sanskrit 'yuj', meaning to yoke or join. But what are the things that we join together? It is the yoking of what you are or what you think you are, with someone up there who is kind of all-powerful. This ancient body of knowledge is not only physical exercise where you twist, turn, bend, stretch and breathe. It is a way of life where you can peer inside your mind and if you get lucky, can also touch your soul!

Activity

Don't let your senses be clouded, spot 'Yoga' in this cloud of words.

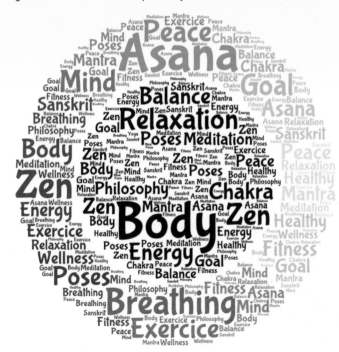

HISTORY OF
YOGA

When and how did Yoga start? Well, what all those wise old men said about Yoga had been written down on palm leaves. But then, palm leaves could be easily damaged, destroyed or lost. So adding a few years here and there, one can roughly claim that Yoga maybe to 10,000 years old. (Quite a long time, eh?) Now, this period can be divided into four main periods.

Pre-Classical Yoga

You first get to hear of Yoga in one of the oldest of the sacred texts of India—the *Rig Veda*. The *Upanishads* taught that you could sacrifice your ego through self-knowledge, action and wisdom. That is real serious stuff.

Classical Yoga

An author of Hindu philosophy called Patanjali, who lived between 2nd century CE to 4th century CE (we do not know the exact dates), wrote the *Yoga-Sutras*. He was an intelligent man and organized the practice of Yoga into an 'eight-limbed path'. This path takes you through the steps and stages towards obtaining Samadhi or enlightenment (but you are not to look out for any halo!).

Post-Classical Yoga

Now, after Patanjali, the Yoga masters decided to reject the teachings of the ancient Vedas. They decided to focus on the physical body and developed Tantra Yoga. This showed you the ways to break the knots that bind you to your physical existence. Another fallout of this rejection was the creation of what you call, the Hatha Yoga.

Modern Yoga

In 1893, Swami Vivekananda from India wowed everyone with his lectures on Yoga at the Parliament of Religions at Chicago. Since then, more Yoga masters traveled to the West and made Hatha or 'wilful' or 'forceful' Yoga quite popular. The Hatha Yoga is a practice of physical Yoga postures and of activity and balance. It is meant to cool you down!

Activity

Can you spot the palm leaf amongst all the leaves on the leaf of this book?

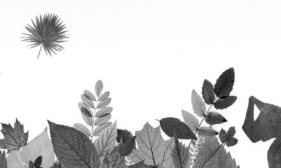

RAJA YOGA

THE PATH OF CONTEMPLATION

The royal one among all the Yogas, Raja Yoga is inclusive of all Yogas and has a philosophy that goes beyond all the others. This Yoga, also known as Mental Yoga, puts emphasis on awareness of the state of mind and the benefits of meditation to get some self-realization, so that the evolution of consciousness happens in a purposeful manner. You learn to calm the mind and focus, through the practice of this Yoga of concentration. Like this, it directs your attention inward, toward your true, divine nature.

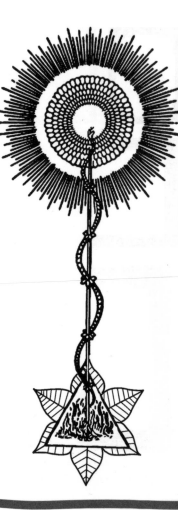

This Yoga plays with your natural powers and trains your mind to be your friend. You are not your mind; you are not your body. Your mind and your body are just "tools" which sometimes work well, while at some, need to be calmed.

This Royal Yoga has an eight-fold path, about which you will get to know later on.

Practicing Raja Yoga gets you to concentrate,
paste eight things that you want to focus on, Mate.

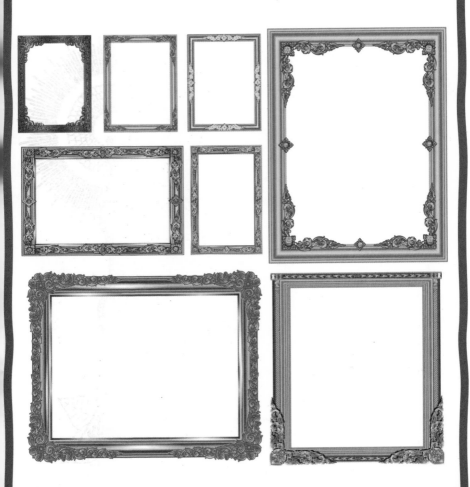

HATHA YOGA

THE PATH OF PHYSICAL TRANSFORMATION

The word "hatha", in most Indian languages, means being adamant. And that is one essential requirement for doing Hatha Yoga—being adamant. When your body and your mind want to give up and say, "We can't do this anymore," you simply be adamant and continue. That for you is Hatha Yoga. Hatha Yoga, by means of intense yogasanas (body postures), will push your physical limitations and make your comfort zone universal. To think about it, how cool would it be! From going beyond your comfort zone and make it universal, you will be at ease wherever you are. Hell won't work for you, you will be adamant enough to frustrate the devil! So, Hatha Yoga makes your body an asset, not a liability, in your progress of becoming ultimate.

In the difficult times that you have been through,
when have you been the most adamant to continue?

_____

_____

_____

_____

_____

_____

_____

_____

_____

_____

_____

_____

_____

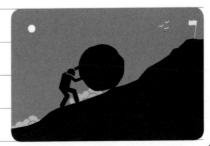

_____

JNANA YOGA

THE PATH OF KNOWLEDGE

Jnana means wisdom or knowledge. So after strengthening the mind and the body, comes the turn of intellect. Jnana Yoga, using intellect as a tool, makes us understand that our true Self is behind and beyond our mind. If you want to become aware of the eternal Self (God), Jnana Yoga is among the best approaches toward that goal. Jnana Yoga takes you on a journey of Self-discovery and probes to ask yourself, "Who am I?" So, you can also call Jnana Yoga the 'Quest for the Self'.

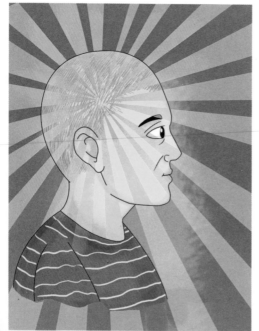

Don't you dare think that Jnana Yoga will be an easy way out, as it requires great strength of will and intellect. Taking you away from "maya" (material thoughts and perceptions) to achieve the union of the "Atman" (inner Self) with the "Brahman" (oneness of all life) is the fundamental aim of Jnana Yoga. So, keep questioning yourself and illuminate yourself.

In the process of questing Self,
analyzing the left and right sides of your brain might help.

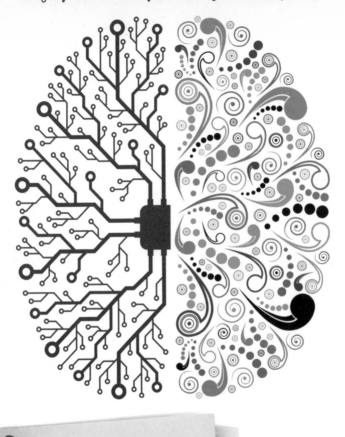

FOUR PILLARS OF
KNOWLEDGE

To open the inner eye, as prescribed by Jnana Yoga, you need to practice the Four Pillars of Knowledge or *Sadhanachatushtaya* (saa-dhu-naa-cha-toosh-taa-ya). But, you need to practice them in a particular order and not when and as you please. They are sure to make you feel less unhappy and less miserable.

1. Viveka (discernment, discrimination) is a continuous, deliberate effort to distinguish between the real and the not-so real, the permanent and the not-so permanent, and the self and the not-so self.

2. Vairagya (detachment) is trying to create non-attachment and indifference toward worldly possessions.

3. Shatsampat (six virtues), as the name suggests, are six mental practices (tranquility, restraint, withdrawal, endurance, faith, focus) to stabilize the mind and emotions and develop the ability to see beyond the illusions of life. Seems like we never fail to take off our rose-tinted glasses!

4. Mumukshutva (longing) is the yearning to achieve liberation from suffering. You need to be completely committed to the path, with such a longing that all other desires fade away.

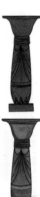
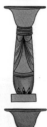
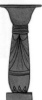

If you had to decide,

what would your four pillars of knowledge look like?

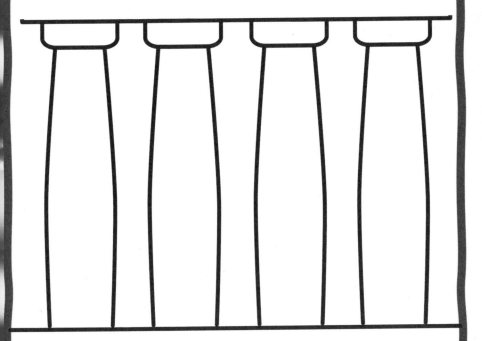

KARMA YOGA
THE PATH OF EGO-FREE ACTION

The word 'karma' means 'to do and to act'. So, any mental or physical act is called karma. Karma Yoga is the Yoga of Action. Now, for all those of you who are of an outgoing nature, this could be your chosen path. But there is a catch. Karma also happens to be the word used to describe the consequences of your action. Whatever your present situation is, it is a result of your past deeds. Likewise, whatever you do now will determine your future. You better watch out, for once you understand this, you can no longer blame anyone else for what happens to you. Sounds a little scary, does it?

There are two types of Karma, Sakama Karma—selfish actions, and Nishkama Karma—selfless actions. Selfish thoughts and actions create a lot of fuss between what is mine and what is yours. Being selfless, however, leads you above and beyond the limit of your little ego.

Karma Yoga, therefore, basically purifies your heart by teaching you to act selflessly, without any thought of gain or reward. By detaching yourself from the fruits of your actions and offering them to God, you learn to sublimate the ego. Poof! And there goes your ego—out of the window. Karma yoga therefore does not allow you to use activity as a means of escape. By insisting that life itself can be holy—it lets you use the tools of everyday life to cut your way to freedom.

Activity

Write down one thing, that you did for someone,
and how did it feel when it was done?

15

BHAKTI YOGA
THE PATH OF LOVE AND DEVOTION

Bhakti (bhuk-ti) Yoga is considered the easiest of all yogic paths—one that would lead you directly to the union of the mind, body and spirit. Bhakti means love and devotion to God—love and devotion to His creation, with respect and care for all living beings and all of Nature—the good, the bad and the ugly. So, a *bhakta* accepts everything that happens to him as a gift of God. There is no desire or expectation, there is simply complete surrender to the will of God. That leaves you absolutely no room for complaining.

The path of Bhakti Yoga appeals particularly to those of an emotional nature.

A person practicing this form of Yoga is motivated chiefly by the power of love and sees God as the embodiment of love. Through prayer, worship and ritual he surrenders himself to God. He channelizes and transmutes his emotions into unconditional love or devotion.

Bhakti Yoga, as the Bhagawad Gita (the religious book of the Hindus) proclaims, is the culmination of other Yoga practices.

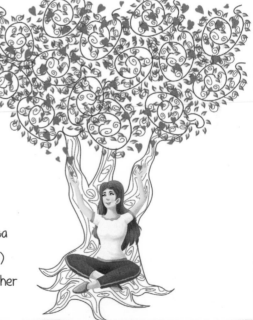

In your heart and mind,

what is the image of the Divine?

THE NINE LIMBS OF
DEVOTION

The ultimate goal in the practice of Bhakti Yoga is to reach the state of *bhakti rasa* (rus) or essence. Bhakti rasa is a feeling of pure bliss achieved when you have given yourself to the divine—lock, stock and barrel. But we cannot attain union with god, without love for all living beings and devotion to God.

To be able to love one and all might seem a difficult proposition. But there are many ways toward developing this path of Bhakti Yoga. There are essentially nine main practices that you could practice independently or together.

A specific *bhava* (bhaav) or feeling, which is suited to different inner constitutions, is created by each of these practices.

1. Shravana (shru-vun)—'listening' to the ancient scriptures, told by a saint or a genuine devotee

2. Kirtana (keer-tun)—'singing' devotional songs

3. Smarana (sma-run)—'remembering' the Divine by meditating upon a name or form

4. Padasevana (pud-se-vun)—'service at the feet' of the Divine

5. Archana (ur-chu-na)—the 'ritual worship' of the Divine

6. Vandana (vun-du-na)—the 'prostration' before the image of the Divine

7. Dasya (das-ya)—the unquestioning devotion and ' serving' of the Divine

8. Sakhya (sakh-ya)—the 'friendship' or the relationship established between the Divine and the devotee

9. Atmanivedana (at-ma-ni-ve-dun)—the 'self-offering' and complete surrender of the self to the Divine

Sit silently for 20 minutes and focus on the Divine,
take inventory of the feelings of your heart while you unwind.

MANTRA YOGA

THE PATH OF POTENT SOUND

The word mantra (mun-tra) comes from the Sanskrit, 'mantrana', meaning suggestion. Mantras are sacred words that, when chanted with concentration and devotion, yield tremendous results on physical, mental and spiritual levels. For example, you could think of the mutterings by witches, wizards or magicians, but of course minus their diabolical connotations.

Mantra Yoga is an exact science where you repeat mantras to gain focus and concentration. The mantras are like warning to tell your mind that it has wandered too far and needs to be back on track. They totally engage your mind and help you get closer to the divinity within you. How soon you are able to achieve concentration depends on the number of times and for how long you can chant the mantras. Chanting doesn't sound bad at all and is good for the one who chants as well as for the one who listens to it.

Through the practice of Mantra Yoga, you can neutralize *rajas* (rujus) or agitation and *tamas* (tumus) or inertia and move into a purer state of consciousness.

They will help to fill the cells of your body with divine energy. They kill the microbes and bring back strength to the cells and tissues. Mantra Yoga in itself is pretty awesome as it improves overall health and mental stability.

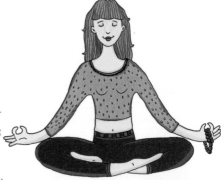

The Gayatri Mantra is the mantra purest of the pure,
find out its meaning for sure.

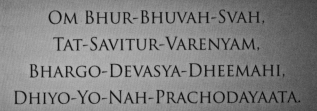

OM BHUR-BHUVAH-SVAH,
TAT-SAVITUR-VARENYAM,
BHARGO-DEVASYA-DHEEMAHI,
DHIYO-YO-NAH-PRACHODAYAATA.

TANTRA YOGA
THE PATH OF CONTINUITY

'Tantra' means to weave or expand. The idea is to weave together many practices of Yoga along with other spiritual styles and teachings, to create a unique way of connecting to the universe. It helps in understanding your body better. Then comes the interesting part. Tantra Yoga helps to improve your sex life as you get in touch with your own body and energy.

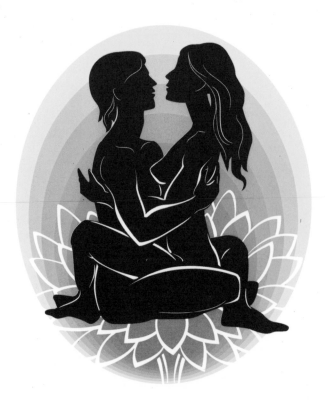

Activity

Tantra Yoga's integral part is sexuality,

join the pieces of this puzzle to make it reach finality.

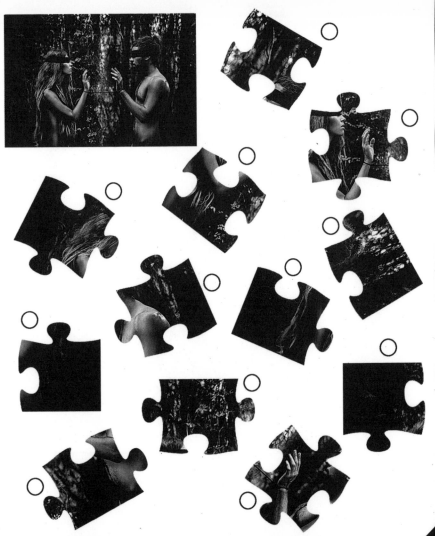

THE EIGHT LIMBS OF
YOGA

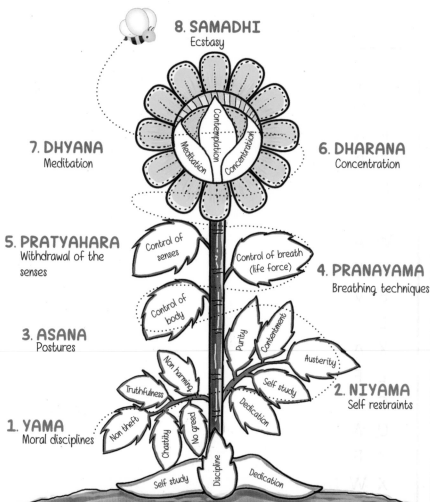

8. SAMADHI
Ecstasy

7. DHYANA
Meditation

6. DHARANA
Concentration

Contemplation

Meditation

Concentration

5. PRATYAHARA
Withdrawal of the senses

Control of senses

Control of breath (life force)

4. PRANAYAMA
Breathing techniques

Control of body

3. ASANA
Postures

Purity

Contentment

Austerity

Non harming

Self study

Truthfulness

Dedication

2. NIYAMA
Self restraints

Non theft

Chastity

No greed

1. YAMA
Moral disciplines

Self study

Discipline

Dedication

The eight limbs of Yoga are right here. Look for them!

```
A Y P D W X M M C D Q I A M P
I M R U J X V G H M I K C A M
P A A I I H D A M A S P N B C
S R N Y V B R O N H H G N L X
H S A D I A G K E I D O N F X
K X Y T N N M E N A Z I K R L
W A A A Y A H R I L U U D Y Y
V Y M Z N A L O F X A U Q X J
B V A A L P H D R C N I Z F M
L J S F E N U A I Z A X M V Y
X A Z H C D O U R Z Y I K F W
L F T Z I K V W T A H D B J V
G T N C Q H U N N E D T F C W
Q W Y A M A K I N Y M K L S U
X B U U J K V Y R T K R K A I
X W H A T Y L F D T J A H T A
```

THE FIVE YAMAS OF
(The five moral disciplines)
YOGA

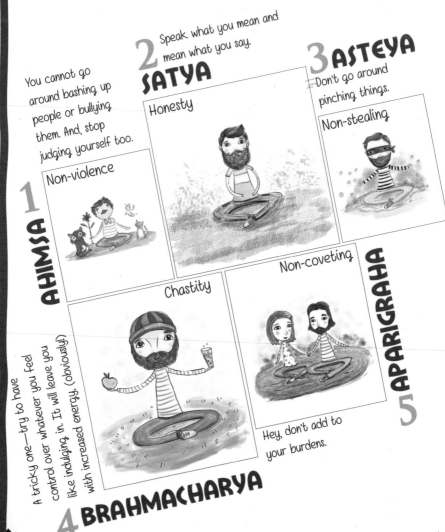

2 SATYA
Speak what you mean and mean what you say.

Honesty

3 ASTEYA
Don't go around pinching things.

Non-stealing

You cannot go around bashing up people or bullying them. And, stop judging yourself too.

Non-violence

1 AHIMSA

Non-coveting

APARIGRAHA 5

Chastity

A tricky one—try to have control over whatever you feel like indulging in. It will leave you with increased energy. (obviously!)

Hey, don't add to your burdens.

4 BRAHMACHARYA

The road to honesty is never an easy one. But nothing that we cannot achieve if we set our minds to it.

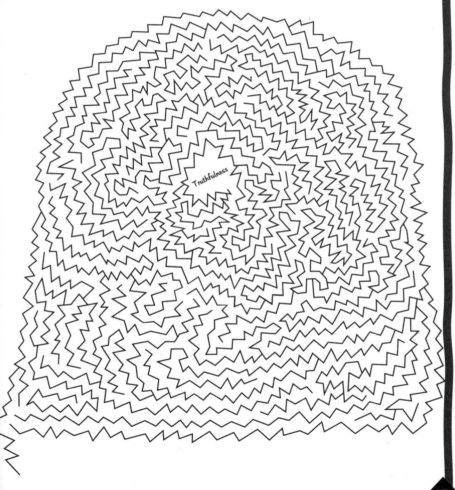

THE FIVE NIYAMAS OF
(The five self-restraints)
YOGA

5 NIYAMAS

SHAUCHA
(purification)

You will become clean inside-out with asana, pranayama and dhyana. You will become strong, too!

SAMTOSHA
(contentment)

You will be happy with what you have and will not cast sidelong glances at what others have.

TAPAS
(asceticism)

Boy, if you manage to master this, you will have perfect control over yourself.

SVADHYAYA
(self-study)

If you think about what all those wise men have said, you will see that you are not a bad one either. There is more to you than what you see in the mirror.

ISHVARA PRANIDHANA
(devotion)

Whatever you have learnt, is, by the way not for yourself. It is for that super being, right up there.

Activity

Now that you know the five niyamas, list five ways in which you can apply them in your life.

ASANAS

(Yoga postures)

Those wise old men of ancient times spent a lot of time sitting and contemplating over things in their minds. Now look, if you choose to spend a lot of time resting on your backside, you would try to be as comfortable as possible. Naturally, asana (posture or pose) in Yoga, literally means to sit. Asanas open your nadis (energy channels) and chakras (psychic centers). They put a brake on you as you run like crazy in your everyday life, and help you focus.

By the way, please don't go over the edge while trying to bend or stretch. Give it your best but there is no need to feel pain, strain or fatigue. And make sure you can breathe slowly and deeply, using Dirga or Ujjaini Pranayama.

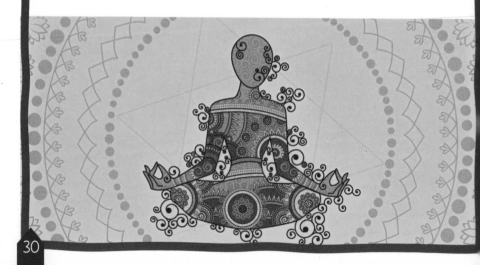

Yoga helps you remember things. Why don't you make a list of things that you would want to remember. Now, focus on them while you do your asanas.

☐ _____
☐ _____
☐ _____
☐ _____
☐ _____
☐ _____
☐ _____
☐ _____
☐ _____
☐ _____
☐ _____
☐ _____
☐ _____
☐ _____
☐ _____
☐ _____

SEATED
YOGA POSTURES

Are you sick and tired of hearing people tell you that you slouch while you sit? Well, you can try out these sitting postures of Yoga. They are quite easy for beginners. Plonking yourself down will not only ground you, but will add to your flexibility.

Energetic Effect: Grounding & Balancing • Physical Effect: Flexibility

PADMASANA

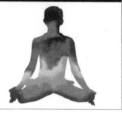

(Lotus)

GOMUKHASANA

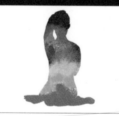

(Cow Face)

HANUMANASANA

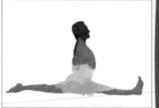

(Monkey)

BALASANA

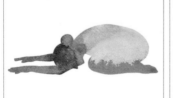

(Child)

PASCHIMOTTANASANA

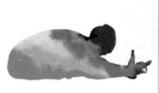

(Seated Forward Bend)

To attain solace, the hands you must trace.

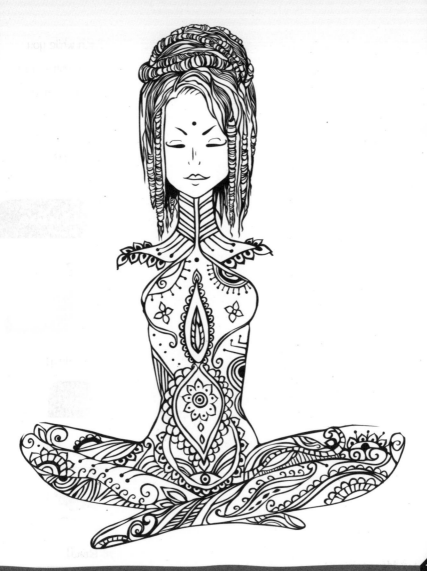

STANDING
YOGA POSTURES

You have to be quite a pro before you try out these. But they go a long way to making you feel healthy, both inside and out. You can do these for shorter times than other poses. They will make you less irritable and help you get back on track.

Energetic Effect: Uplifting & Opening • Physical Effect: Strength

GARUDASANA
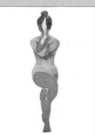
(Eagle)

UTTHITA TRIKONASANA
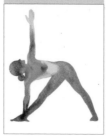
(Triangle)

UTTANASANA
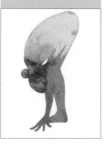
(Forward Bend)

VIBHADRASANA
(Warrior)

DANDAYAMANA DHANURASANA
(Bow Pulling)

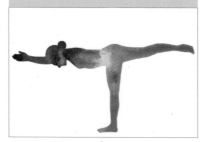
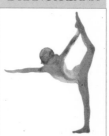

Can you identify the standing Yoga postures?

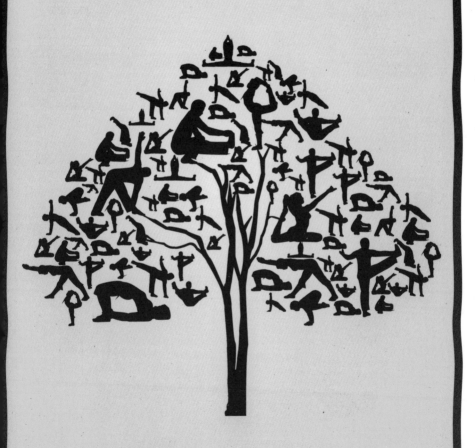

PRONE
YOGA POSTURES

Don't go by the look of these poses. Though easy enough for beginners, they can be quite tough to hold on for longer periods. They are bound to make you feel energetic, loaded and ready to go.

Energetic Effect: Energizing • Physical Effect: Back & Core Strength

SHALABHASANA

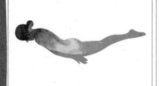

(Locust)

URDHVA MUKHA SVANASANA

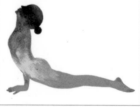

(Upward-Facing Dog)

SALAMBA BHUJANGASANA

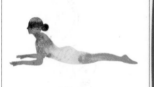

(Sphinx)

ASHTANGASANA

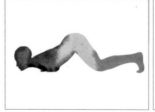

(Eight Limbed)

SARVANGASANA

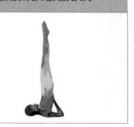

(Shoulder Stand)

Prone Yoga poses help you lose that extra weight. How much have you managed to lose in two months? Color this perfect body to motivate yourself.

DAY 1	DAY 15	DAY 30	DAY 45	DAY 60

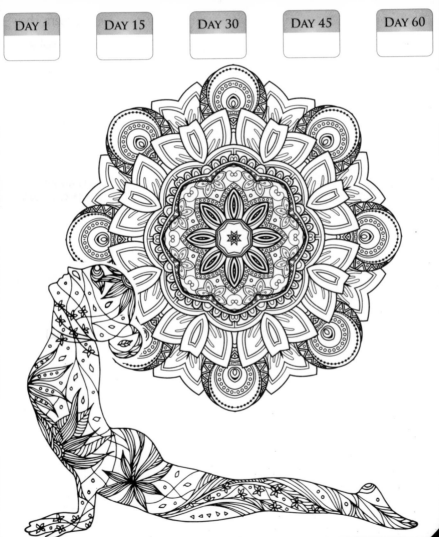

SUPINE
YOGA POSTURES

Supine Yoga postures are done on your back and are a great way to end your Yoga practice. Supine postures release stress, promote flexibility, and help to sum up your practice.

Energetic Effect: Nurturing & Integrating • Physical Effect: Flexibility

HALASANA

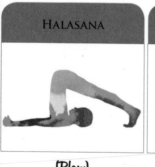

(Plow)

MATSYASANA

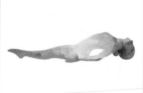

(Fish)

SUPTA MATSYENDRASANA

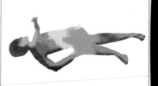

(Knee Down Twist)

PAVANAMUKTASAN

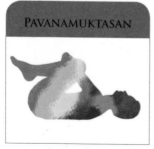

(Wind Relieving)

SHAVASANA

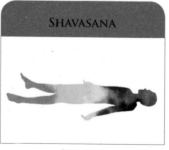

(Corpse)

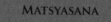

A Yoga posture that is supine, will appear when you join the dots with lines, fine.

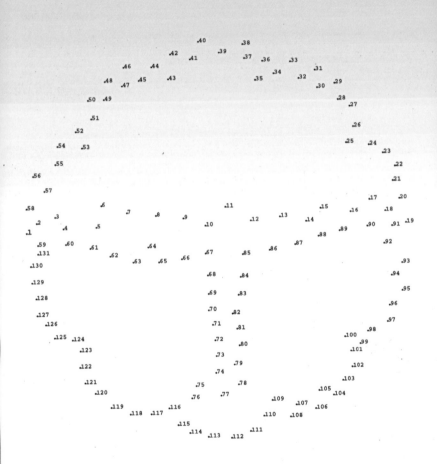

PRANAYAMA

(Breathing techniques)

'Prana' (praan) plus 'ayama' (aayum) make up 'pranayama' (praanayum).

'Prana' is 'vital energy' or 'life force'—the force that runs through all things around you. 'Ayama' is 'extension', or 'expansion' of 'prana'—in other words, extension or expansion of the dimension of 'prana'.

Now, the pranayama exercise make use of your breathing to make the life force flow through the nadis or energy channels of your body. This way, you can go beyond your normal boundaries or limitations and feel quite like a superhero with a higher state of vibratory energy.

Now, time for some technicalities. In pranayama practices, there are four important aspects of breathing:

1. Pooraka (Pu-ra-k) – inhalation—taking in air

2. Rechaka (Re-cha-k) – exhalation—giving out air

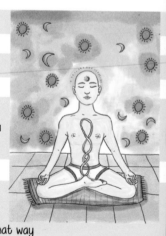

3. Antarkumbhaka (Antur-koom-bha-k) – internal breath retention—this is tricky—holding your breath when you have taken in air and your lungs are full

4. Bahir kumbhaka (Baa-hir koom-bha-k) – external breath retention—this is when you have given out air and your lungs are empty and you try to keep them that way

These practices of pranayama, especially antarakumbhaka, calm you down. Stillness of breath leads to stillness of mind.

When you will do,

how will pranayama benefit you?

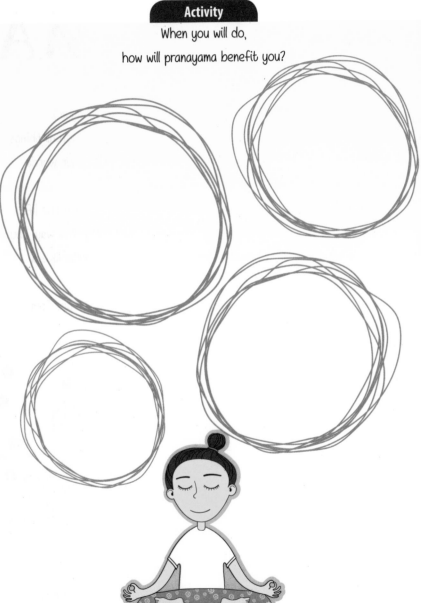

PRANIC BODY

The human framework, you would be surprised to know, is made up of five koshas or sheaths:

1. Annamaya kosha – the food or material body—the five elements
2. Pranamaya kosha – the bioplasmic or the vital energy body—the five pranas
3. Manomaya kosha – the mental body or the outer mind
4. Vijnanamaya kosha – the higher mental body or intelligence
5. Anandamaya kosha – the transcendental body or memory, subliminal and superconscious mind

The Pranamaya Kosha, consisting of our vital life energies, sort of balances between the physical body on one side and the three sheaths of the mind on the other. A person with a strong vital nature, becomes prominent in life but can end up being a bully too. Interestingly, a powerful Pranamaya Kosha is also important for the spiritual path—but this kind of vital force derives strength not from personal power but from humility and complete surrender to the Divine.

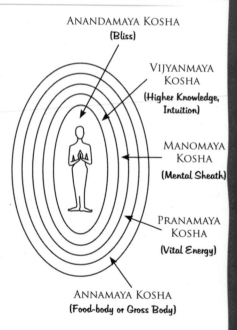

ANANDAMAYA KOSHA
(Bliss)

VIJYANMAYA KOSHA
(Higher Knowledge, Intuition)

MANOMAYA KOSHA
(Mental Sheath)

PRANAMAYA KOSHA
(Vital Energy)

ANNAMAYA KOSHA
(Food-body or Gross Body)

To strengthen your Pranic body, doing pranayama is the key,
name all the pranayams you would want to do, sitting by the sea.

FIVE PRANAS

This all-important Pranamay Kosha is made up of five Pranas.

1. Prana – This is all about the force by which you take in air inside your body. In the process, it also regulates anything that you intake—be it food, drinks or emotions.

2. Apana – This is exactly the opposite of Prana, being the guiding force of things that are thrown out of your body. It is the expulsion of all waste products including hurtful feelings, sentiments and emotions.

3. Udana – You will be surprised to know that this helps you stand and grow and also does a lot for

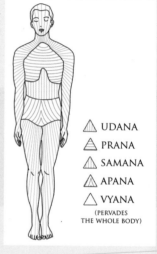

△ UDANA
△ PRANA
△ SAMANA
△ APANA
△ VYANA
(PERVADES THE WHOLE BODY)

your will and enthusiasm. Without it, you would not be half as conscious about the outside world and might end up being a zombie.

4. Samana – This is what helps you keep your balance. It helps you get over your hangovers, helps in digestion of food, and helps you to digest experiences, in other words, it helps you take life in your stride.

5. Vyana – It controls circulation on all levels. It moves the food, water and oxygen and also your feelings and emotions, throughout your body. Thank god it does, as this movement gives you power and strength. This also lets the other Pranas do their work.

Psychologically, Prana and Apana together help us to stay positive,
Make your way toward losing all the negativity so addictive.

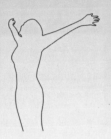

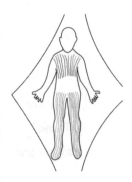

PRATYAHARA

(Withdrawal of the Senses)

You have often heard about putting yourself in somebody else's shoes. How about putting yourself in a turtle's shell? If you were to be a turtle and would withdraw into your shell, how would you feel? Pratyahara comes from 'prati' meaning 'against' or 'away' and 'ahara' meaning 'food' or 'anything we take into ourselves from the outside'. So, pratyahara is not only letting go of those mouth-watering snacks, but also being able to control all external influences. It is about opening up to the right impressions and associations. The turtle's shell is the mind and its limbs are the senses. By withdrawing the sensory impressions, the mind is free to move within.

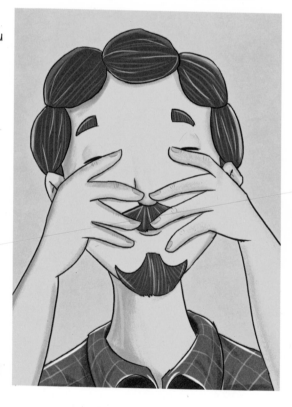

While getting away from the influences of life,

getting away from which you strife?

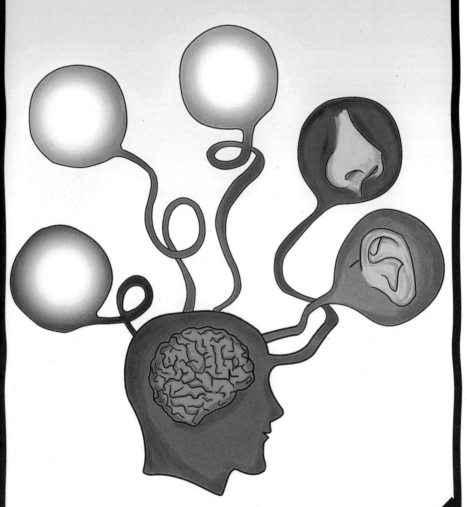

DHARANA

(Concentration)

Dharana, the sixth limb of Yoga, is 'concentration'. By concentration, you are not meant to stare blankly. Rather, you are free to choose the place where you would like to place your awareness and attention. Swami Vivekananda had said that the mind is 'a drunken monkey'. (Monkeys are of no good, and drunken ones at that must be a real nuisance!) So it is basically about

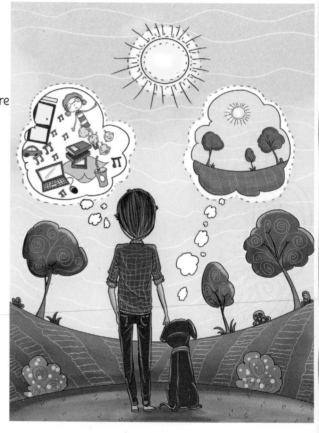

getting hold of your 'monkey mind' and then bringing it back to whatever you are focusing on. Again, and again, and again.

Concentration is the way to go,
concentrate and get out of this brain maze, like a pro.

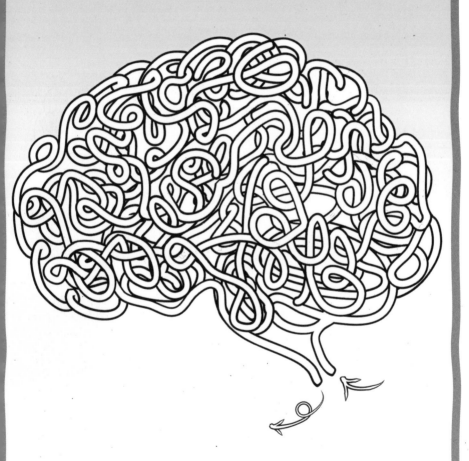

DHYANA

(Meditation)

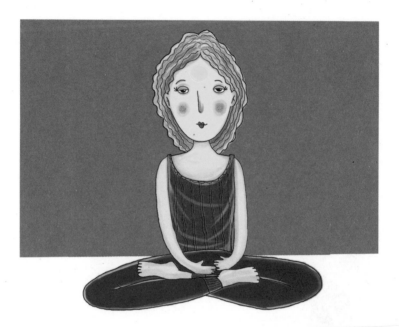

The seventh limb of Yoga is only a build-up upon the practices of asana, pranayama, pratyahara, and dharana. It is all about tackling not only your mind, but also your senses. So, you need to cut the supply routes that carry sensations to the brain constantly during wakefulness, sleep, and dreams. Then, you need to focus on a point—it could be a yellow flower, the corner of your sofa, a white dog, a light, a star or anything of your heart's desire. When your mind is fully detached, you are so caught up in the act that you will feel yourself to be a part of the process itself!

When you practice dhyana, what do you want to tackle?

As you climb each ladder, you face which obstacle?

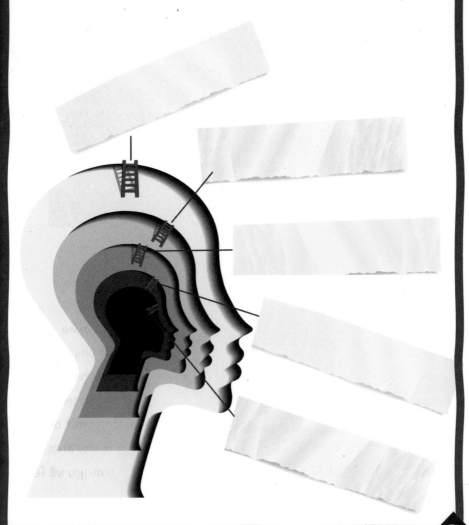

SAMADHI
(Ecstacy)

Samadhi is quite serious stuff and not something that you can achieve at one go. 'Sama' means equanimity and 'dhi' means 'buddhi' or the intellect. So, if you reach an equanimous state of the intellect, it is known as samadhi. An equanimous state is one in which you transcend your intellect. Now, this does not mean that you become foolish or insane. It means that you are no longer limited by your senses—time and space do not exist for you. You become one with reality—what is here is there, what is now is then. Sounds quite like something out of a sci-fi film, does it not?

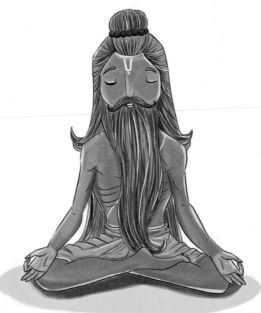

When you reach the equanimous state of intellect,

what in your mind does reflect?

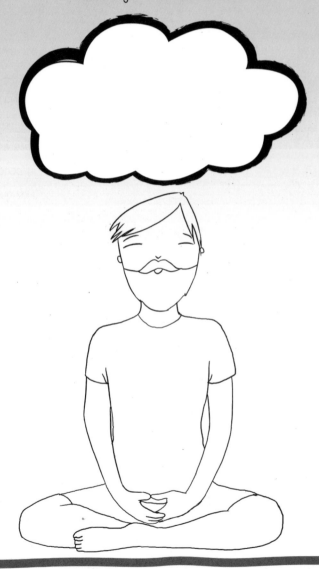

THE SEVEN
CHAKRAS

There are 114 chakras associated to human body. There are many more than that but these are the major ones. You can see them as junction boxes or merging points of nadis. They are referred to as 'chakras', meaning wheels or circles, because they embody movement from one dimension to another. In reality, they are triangles. Of these 114, two happen to be outside the body. Of the remaining 112, only 108 can be worked upon. Hence, the number 108, holds great significance in spiritual practices.

The seven basic chakras are more commonly known as the chakra system. These are the energy centers that are constantly in motion along the human spinal column. Each possessing its own color and vibrational frequency, the chakras act as the catalysts of consciousness and human function. Various emotional issues, from survival instincts and self-esteem to the ability to communicate and experience love are governed by chakras.

Chakra balancing makes for a large part of getting to know how to work with chakras since a chakra blockage in one or more of these seven chakras can initiate mental, emotional, physical or spiritual ailments.

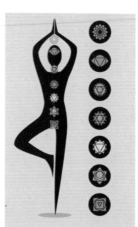

SAHASRARA

AJNA

VISHUDDHA

ANAHATA

MANIPURA

SVADHISTHANA

MULADHARA

There are seven basic chakras,

find their names in this word search—don't let it pass.

E	E	R	J	X	N	C	R	I	Q	Q	V	T	X	A	B	L	H	C	Q
G	E	O	V	A	Q	M	Q	P	V	M	V	A	T	N	G	D	U	U	O
Y	Y	Q	I	W	P	F	M	C	J	K	V	Z	A	M	Q	I	S	J	B
E	V	V	Q	R	W	J	F	R	G	I	A	T	L	S	K	U	L	K	Y
H	D	J	T	S	S	V	A	D	H	I	S	T	H	A	N	A	W	A	A
Z	K	V	S	K	S	E	A	J	R	K	P	Q	J	B	P	H	U	S	O
K	W	R	Z	E	F	R	U	A	F	Y	Q	I	C	V	Z	D	R	W	X
A	D	M	B	F	U	Q	H	S	N	N	K	J	D	L	X	D	Y	X	N
R	N	H	X	P	U	Z	R	C	F	J	R	R	Y	T	N	U	M	Q	A
K	A	U	I	J	Y	K	T	W	X	E	A	S	I	Q	T	H	Q	I	T
N	N	N	T	Y	X	N	Y	X	W	G	A	G	T	I	I	S	N	G	M
C	A	W	C	N	E	Y	O	F	A	K	C	E	M	L	I	I	S	T	W
M	H	W	Z	V	X	P	Z	E	A	W	V	A	U	E	J	V	K	R	C
Y	A	V	T	F	U	A	F	L	X	X	I	H	L	Q	M	W	H	C	U
M	T	E	I	T	P	S	R	A	G	S	A	H	A	S	R	A	R	A	G
S	A	S	Y	Z	W	Z	S	M	C	D	A	S	D	J	C	Q	U	B	O
J	R	T	E	P	N	X	B	A	X	C	H	L	H	N	J	I	Y	G	P
K	S	N	G	P	O	I	K	N	Z	H	M	T	A	U	Q	P	B	M	U
F	S	V	D	X	I	W	A	W	Q	L	V	K	R	Y	E	E	O	S	M
A	K	L	F	Z	U	G	X	I	Q	T	W	E	A	C	E	I	B	X	O

MULADHARA

ROOT CHAKRA

Element – earth   Color – red

Muladhara (mool-aa-dha-ra) is located at the perineum, the space between the anal outlet and the genital organ. Muladhara is really made up of two terms: 'moola' means the root or source, and 'adhar' means the foundation. It is the foundation of the energy body.

Muladhar connects to your grounded-ness and instincts of survival and governs your family ties, belonging and guardedness. You can find your earliest memories stored here. And if the foundation is unstable, anxiety is natural.

If Muladhara goes off-balance or gets blocked, you can become needy, have low self-esteem or self-destructive behaviors. But when Muladhara is in balance, it makes you feel strong and confident—you can stand up on your feet and take care of yourself.

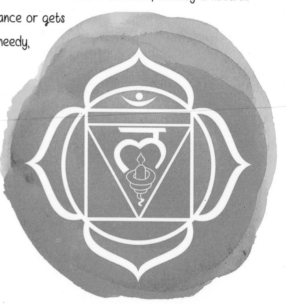

Muladhara caters to the roots of life,

join the dots to make its symbol, in minutes less than five.

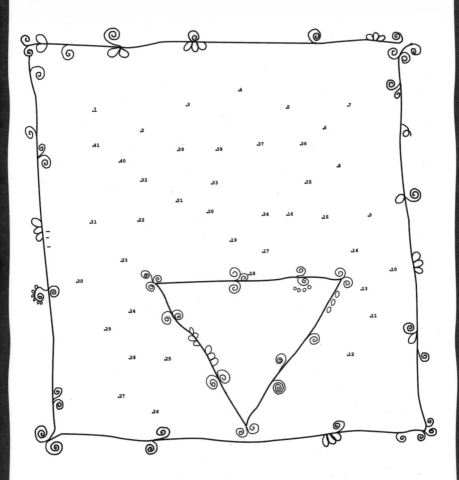

SWADHISTHANA
SACRAL OR PELVIC CHAKRA

Element – water   Color – orange

Swadhisthana (swa-dhi-sh-tha-na) is located just above the genital organ. In accordance with its location, this chakra corresponds with your reproductive and sexual organs and represents fluidity, creativity and fertility. If your energies happen to move into Swadhisthana, you are a pleasure seeker. When this chakra is active, you enjoy the physical world in a lot of ways. Looking at a pleasure seeker, you can see that his life and his experience of life are just a little more intense compared with a person who is only about food and sleep. You can interpret this, or associate this chakra with whether or not you feel deserving of a pleasurable, abundant, creative life. When this chakra goes out of balance, you feel emotionally unstable, guilty, or hard on yourself. When Swadhisthana is in balance, you feel creative, positive, and receptive to change—you're in the flow, like the ocean and its tides.

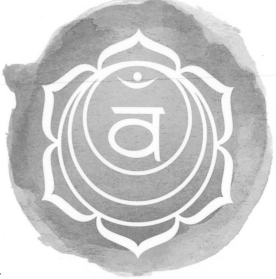

Swadhisthana corresponds to fluidity,
write about when you felt the least and the most of it.

_____

_____

_____

_____

_____

_____

_____

_____

_____

_____

_____

_____

_____

_____

_____

_____

MANIPURA

NAVEL CHAKRA

Element – fire   Color – yellow

Manipura (mani-pu-rah) is located just below the navel. It connects to your ego, will and, personal power and autonomy. If your energy moves into the Manipura, you are a doer in the world. You are all about action and can do many, many things. When Manipura is balanced, you feel alive and have the self-confidence and esteem to take actions and get your productivity into full swing.

But when it gets blocked, you face adverse effects—you lack courage, have low self-confidence and esteem and feel stagnant and incapable. You can awaken your true personal inner power by focusing on this chakra and also overcome your fear of taking risks.

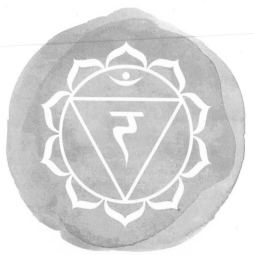

Manipura rules your doing and action,
complete the symbol below, don't ask for a reason.

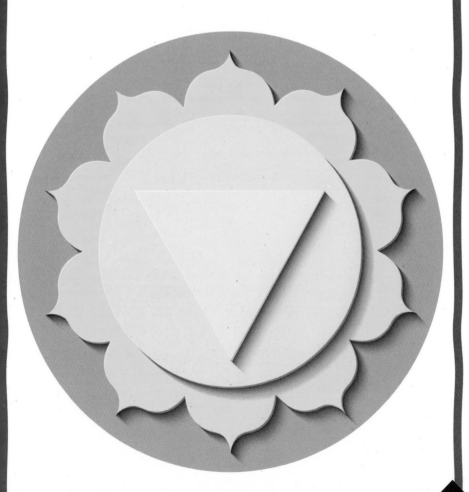

ANAHATA
HEART CHAKRA

Element – air   Color – green

The three lower chakras are mainly concerned with your physical existence. Anahata (ana-ga-da) is a combination—it is a meeting place for both the survival and the enlightenment chakras. The word *Anahata* literally means the 'un-struck'. The three lower Anahatas is located in the heart area and acts as a transition between your lower and higher chakras.

Anahata awakens the power of unconditional love within you through compassion, forgiveness and acceptance. When this chakra gets blocked, you become pretty possessive and codependent and may form dysfunctional relationships. It brings a fear of rejection and makes you isolated. By stimulating this one, you can work wonders and heal past wounds, learn to love unconditionally and form happy, healthy relationships.

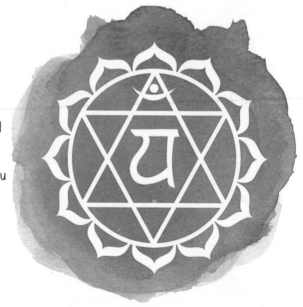

Anhata rules the heart,
make its symbol, joining every part.

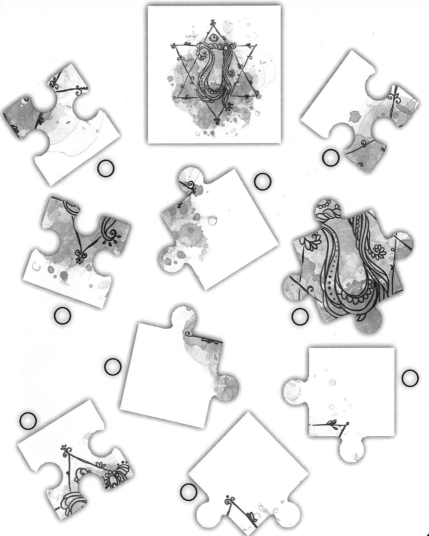

VISHUDDHA
THROAT CHAKRA

Element – ether   Color – blue

Vishuddha (vi-shoo-dha) is located in the area of your throat. Vishuddha literally means 'filter'. If your energies happen to move into this chakra, you become a very powerful human being, in many ways. Power is not only political or administrative—you can become so powerful that even if you just sit in one place, things will happen for you on their own. Interesting, this sounds. When Vishuddha gets blocked, it can make you feel you can't find your voice or your truth. You can become overly talkative and not listen to others. But your voice moves through space to help you communicate your emotions in healthy ways, when this chakra is open and stimulated. It also makes you a better listener and helps you understand others better.

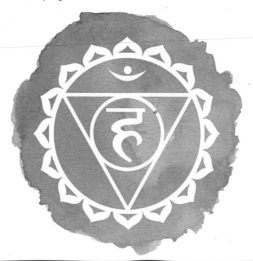

Vishuddha governs your understanding and gives you voice,
write about an issue close to your heart, of your choice.

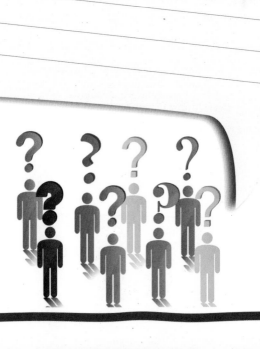

AJNA
THIRD-EYE CHAKRA

Element – light   Color – indigo

Ajna (aag-na) is located between your eyebrows. If your energies happen to move to this chakra, you become intellectually enlightened. This chakra corresponds with your intuition, or sixth sense, and governs how the rest of the chakras function. When Ajna is well stimulated, it gives you insight and makes you trust your inner wisdom to face life's challenges and choices. This must be the one that the detectives are so fond of.

It makes you attain a new balance and peace inside yourself. When it's blocked, it can make you cynical, close-minded, over attached to logic and also give you trust issues. In order to open your mind to the bigger picture and different perspectives, work on this chakra. It also helps you receive the wisdom that cannot be seen or heard by ordinary senses.

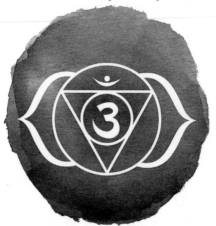

Ajna represents the third eye,
color it bright and high you fly!

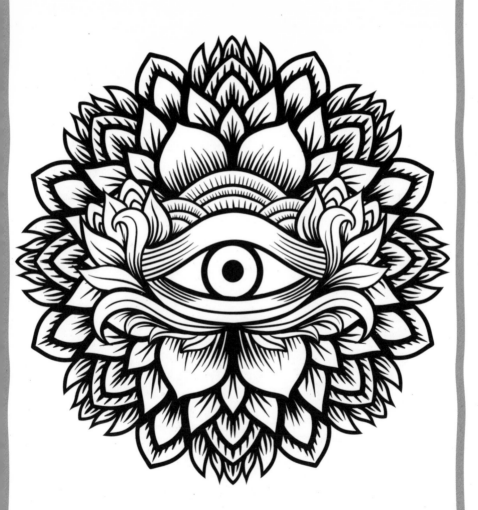

SAHASRARA

CROWN CHAKRA

Element – cosmic energy   Color – violet

Saharara (sahas-ra-ra) is located at the top, or at the crown of your head. It directly corresponds to beauty (better take care of it) and to the spiritual realm. This chakra gives you an insight and helps you understand who you are beyond your physical self.

It tells you that you are in fact a spiritual being in human garb. It actually hovers above the crown of the head and not located inside the body. When it's closed, it makes you suffer by putting in the thought that happiness can only come from the outside.

If you work on this chakra, it will help you feel free in any situation. If your energies happens to move into Sahasrara, you become kind of ecstatic beyond all reason, bursting with ecstasy for no reason whatsoever. (Not a very good idea to try it!)

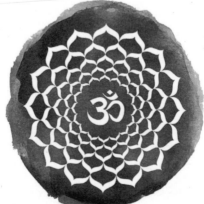

In the human body structure,

mark the position of Sahasrara and all the others.

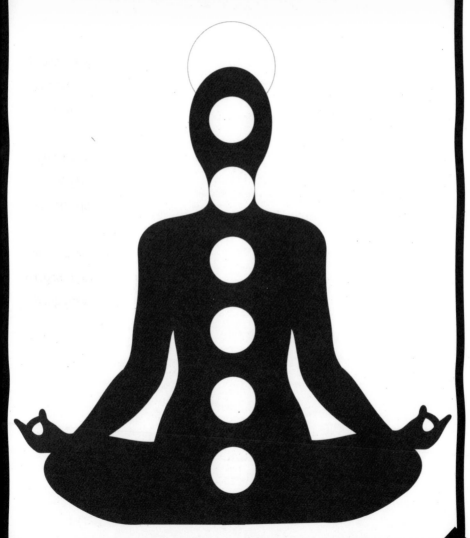

(The Yoga of Awareness)
KUNDALINI
THE MOST DANGEROUS FORM

Kundalini (kun-da-li-ni) is an ancient Sanskrit word that literally means 'coiled snake'. Long, long ago, in early Eastern religion, it was believed that each individual possessed a divine energy at the base of the spine. (Is this the reason that the chill we feel is always at the bottom of the spine?) This energy was thought to be the sacred energy of creation. Although we are born with this energy, we need to make a conscious effort to 'uncoil the snake', and that too for our own benefit. Uncoiling the snake would put us in direct contact with the divine. As the 'Yoga of awareness', the philosophical purpose of Kundalini is to awaken your higher divine self.

In its essence, Kundalini is the most dangerous form of Yoga, as it is also the most potent. What is most potent is almost always the most dangerous if improperly handled. Saying this does not, in any way mean that there is something wrong with Kundalini Yoga. It's just that that it needs to be guided properly. You can make or burn your life out of it. Energy has no discretion of its own, it is how you use it. In order to activate Kundalini, you need to prepare the body, mind and emotion because it pumps out huge volumes of energy into the system.

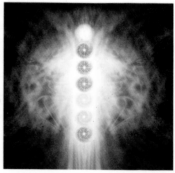

Snakes scare some, some are scared of spaces closed,

what gives you chills, if exposed?

KUNDALINI YOGA

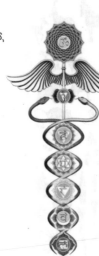

Like a coiled-up snake that is very hard to see till it moves, the nature of Kundalini is such that when it is still, you won't even know of its existence. It's only when it moves that you realize there is so much power within yourself. If your kundalini happens to get aroused, things that you never imagined to be possible—miraculous things—will happen with you.

No matter what you do, the whole Yogic system is aimed only toward enhancing your perception. You only know what you perceive. Heightened states of energy are also heightened states of perception. This is why the symbolism of the Hindu God Shiva and a snake is used. It indicates that his energies have reached the peak and thus, his third eye has opened.

The third eye means another dimension of perception in a human being has opened up. The two eyes are limited to seeing that is physical but the third eye opens another dimension of perception altogether.

Kundalini Yoga is performed by imagining yourself to move in an anti-clockwise direction. This results in unwinding the Kundalini that rises upward from the root chakra.

Kundalini is represented by a snake,

find one here, try hard for Kundalini's sake.

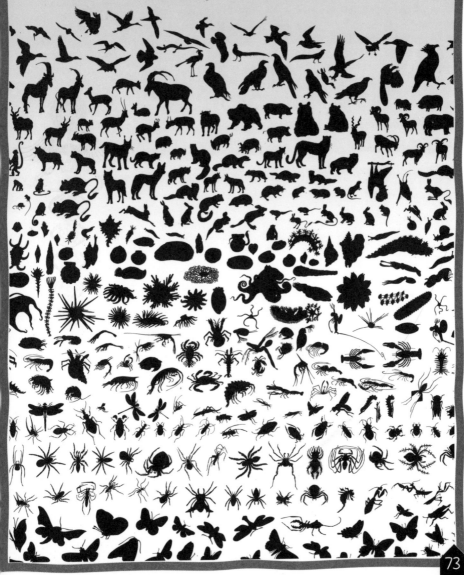

73

GURU

(The teacher)

Guru is the Sanskrit word for teacher—'gu' means darkness and 'ru' means dispeller. Thus, guru is the dispeller of darkness. Quite an important one, that one is—he is the one who diverts you from the path of *avidya* (ignorance) to *vidya* (knowledge). He will not stuff you with knowledge (thank god for that), but arouse your intelligence.

He will show you who you are and what is your highest possibility. He works to remove the veil from your spirituality so that you attain clarity of thought and sight.

The guru passes on *parampara* or knowledge in its most genuine, authenticate form to his disciples. So never miss out on any teaching from your guru.

The guru is presence unlimited—vast, infinite and all-inclusive. He is God incarnate and the doorway to liberation. In other words, God, Guru and Self are synonymous.

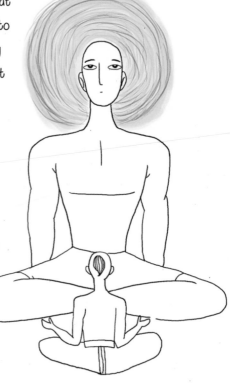

Home, school, work or wherever,
what's your fondest memory with a teacher?

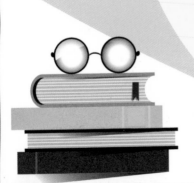

BENEFITS OF
YOGA

As you have been reading and going through this book, you must have realized that Yoga has innumerable benefits—physical, emotional, spiritual and more. It's always a win-win situation when it comes to Yoga (obviously only if you practice it right). Let's look at some of them as Yoga:

1. improves your flexibility and builds your muscle strength (so no need sweat it out at the gym)

2. perfects your posture and protects your spine

3. prevents cartilage and joint breakdown

4. improves the health of your bones

5. increases blood flow

6. boosts your immunity by draining your lymph cells

7. relieves depression and makes you happier

8. helps you get rid of high blood pressure and blood sugar

9. regulates your adrenal glands

10. helps you focus and relaxes your system

Activity

In all the times you have been blue,

how has Yoga helped you?

11. improves your balance

12. maintains your nervous system

13. gets you good sleep

14. gives your lungs space to breathe

15. prevents digestive issues

16. provides peace of mind

17. increases your self-esteem

18. gives you inner strength and soothes your pain

19. keeps you away from drug addiction

20. makes you alert and aware

21. leads to healthy relationships

22. cures many ailments

23. keeps allergies and viruses away from you

24. encourages self-care and helps you serve others

25. heals you and helps you change

Look left and right and up and down,

write all the ways Yoga can help you around.

SURYA
NAMASKAR
(Sun Salutations)

Ah! The hands always reaching out to the snooze-mode syndrome. Salute the sungod and warm up for the day. These Yoga poses will work wonders with your body. You will feel positive energy flow through you and tingle all your senses.

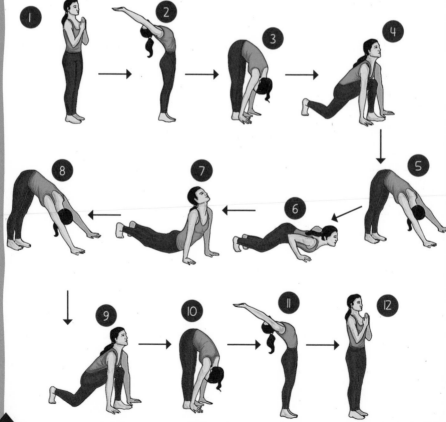

1. Ashwa Sanchalanasana (equestrian)

2. Bhujangasana (cobra)

3. Pranamasana (prayer)

4. Padahastasana (hand to foot)

5. Ashtangasana (eight limbed)

6. Hasta Utthanasana (raised arms)

7. Parvatasana (mountain)

Here are the names of the seven asanas of Suryanamaskar. Arrange them in the order in which they should be performed.

1. _____

2. _____

3. _____

4. _____

5. _____

6. _____

7. _____

CHANDRA
NAMASKAR
(Moon Salutations)

The Moon, as you know, doesn't have its own light and reflects the light of the Sun. Similarly, the Chandra Namaskar or the Moon salutations are nothing but a reflection of the Sun salutations. Most of the postures, you see, are just the same. Moon salutations are best practiced at night, in the presence of the Moon (obviously!). Also, make sure your stomach is empty when you do these. Moon salutations channelize the lunar energy that has cool, relaxing and creative qualities. These asanas help you relax, calm down, and get your creative horses running.

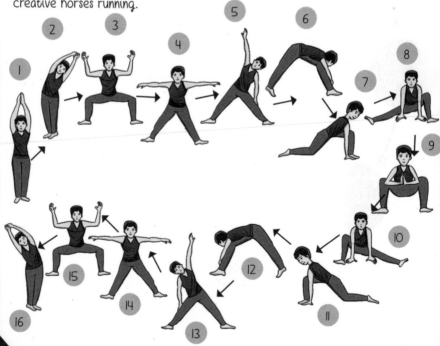

It's not-so soon,

for you to name the phases of the moon.

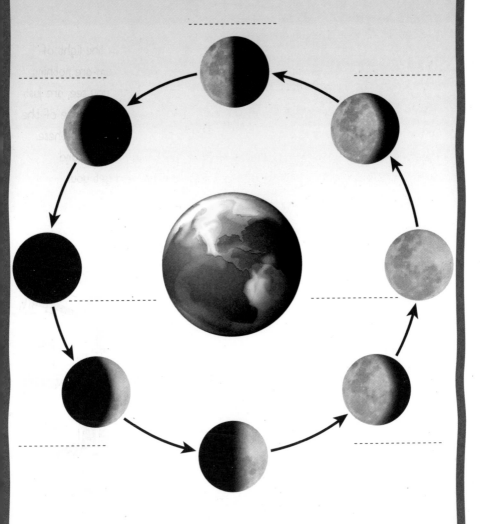

WHEN YOUR MIND SAYS TOMORROW

According to a popular Indian superstition, as the Sun sets, villagers get scared of the fact that demons might appear. To prevent that from happening, they paint a sign that means 'come tomorrow', on their doors. It is a signal for the demons to come the next day. But as the tomorrow never comes, the demons do not come too. Sounds like a great idea, doesn't it?

Tomorrow is always a better day. But to really do what you intend on doing, you need to tune your body to what is there in your mind.

If you plan on waking up early to do Yoga, but eat an entire pizza late at night, your body will simply ask you to go back to sleep at dawn. But if you eat light and early, your body will awaken at dawn and you will be fresh to do Yoga. You have to set a resolve and create the necessary ambience to do what is needed. If you create a proper atmosphere for doing something, you will be eager to do it.

Tomorrow has to be created today and as a popular Indian couplet states, do

tomorrow's work today, today's work now. If the moment gets lost, how will the work be done? Do the work that needs to be done, now. There is no better time than NOW.

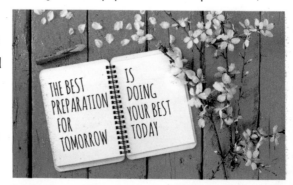

THE BEST PREPARATION FOR TOMORROW IS DOING YOUR BEST TODAY

Activity

The mind might ask you to put it on tomorrow,
but finish this sudoku today as you go.

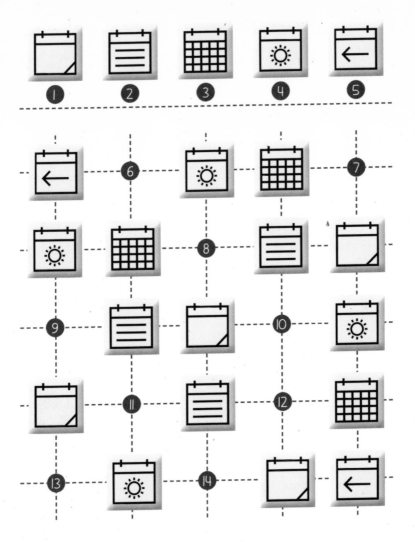

YOGA FADS

These days, so many people are practicing Yoga that if taken all together, they could perhaps form an entire continent. And as it happens, when so many people are involved in something, bizarre things happen. So with Yoga. Many different forms of Yoga have come up. Some of them are so strange that they actually tax the imagination. So ready for a few surprises?

Nude Yoga – As the name suggests, you will be naked. Yes, in a class full of people!

Aerial Yoga – Taking Yoga practice to new heights, quite literally!

Paddleboard Yoga – Imagine keeping your balance on water!

Doga – Doga or Dog Yoga! Get your furry friends along!

Cannabis Yoga – One for all the recreational pot lovers!

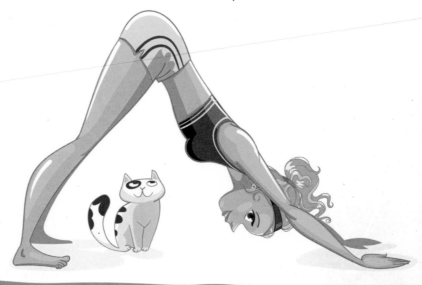

Activity

Take part,
and make your own Yoga fad card.

BEER YOGA

Among all the fads that have built up around Yoga, this is the most popular one. Beer Yoga originated in Germany as 'the marriage of two great lovers—beer and Yoga'. Both the practices are centuries old and combining them together is fun, but no joke. It is for beer lovers who like Yoga and for Yogis who like beer. So, when are you picking up a glass to try this?

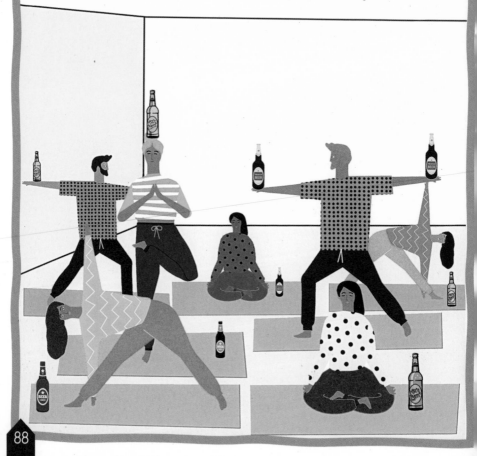

Yoga and drinks are two necessities in life,

write your choice of drinks, for which you strife.

YOGA
AT HOME

Have you also been in those situations when you are all pumped up about watching DVDs, learning, and then doing Yoga at home, all on your own? And did it ever work out? Ah, we know how it feels. Just stick to it, maybe, just maybe, it will work out (umm, you will work out).

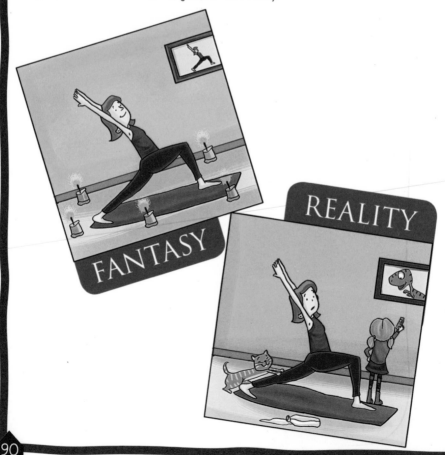

Day in, day out,

draw what your Yoga practice is about.

SELF-PRACTICE

I can do it! Or can I? I am doing it right! Or am I?

When you start doing Yoga (that is, if you stop planning and actually start doing it), innumerable thoughts will cross your head. But to beat it all, and to be true to the spirit of it, stick to it. Try a little harder each day. Who knows what miracles might await you!?

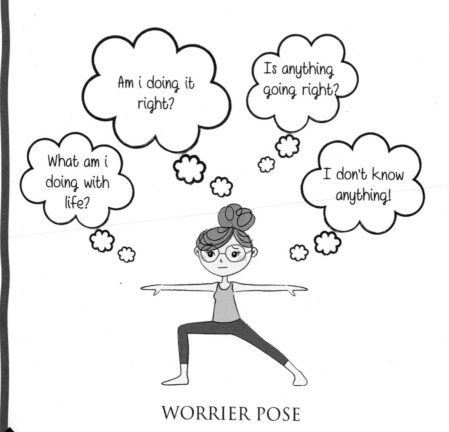

WORRIER POSE

Activity

Some Yoga poses here have been shown,
give them a name, of your own.

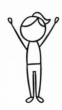 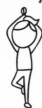 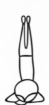 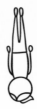 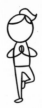

- - - - - - - -   - - - - - - - -   - - - - - - - -   - - - - - - - -   - - - - - - - -

- - - - - - - -   - - - - - - - -   - - - - - - - -   - - - - - - - -   - - - - - - - -

- - - - - - - -   - - - - - - - -   - - - - - - - -   - - - - - - - -

- - - - - - - -   - - - - - - - -   - - - - - - - -   - - - - - - - -

NAMASTE
THE SIMPLEST FORM OF YOGA

The word 'Namaste' breaks down to 'nama' meaning bow, 'as' meaning I and 'te' meaning you. So, it literally means, 'I bow to you'. This is one of the ways of greeting in India and the perfect way to end this book.

Yoga classes or any Yoga practice ends when you fold your hands at the position of the heart chakra and do a Namaste to your teacher. Ideally, it should be done in the beginning but it is done at the end because the atmosphere in the room is serene and peaceful, and in sync with the universe. The Namaste is initiated by the teacher to show gratitude and respect toward her students and to her own teachers. This, in turn, invites the student to follow the lineage and to allow the truth to flow.

For a teacher and student, Namaste thus allows them to come together as two individuals to a place of connection and timelessness, free from the bonds of ego-connection. If it is done with deep feeling in the heart and with the mind surrendered, a deep union of spirits can blossom.

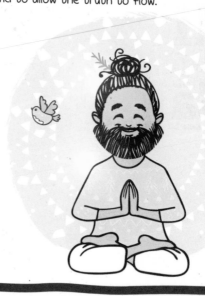